TABLE OF CONTENTS

INTRODUCTION

CHAPTER 1

PRACTICE GOOD CONSUMING HABIT

Chapter 2

WEIGHT LOSS TIPS

Chapter 3

SUCCESSFUL WEIGHT LOSS TIPS

Chapter 4

STAY POSITIVE

DISCLAIMER

INTRODUCTION

It is normal to feel worried when trying to lose weight because you need to figure out how to eat healthily and fuel your body correctly, create a diet and exercise routine that works for you, get plenty of sleep, and sooner or later make thousands of choices every day that will either bring you closer to your goal or throw you completely off track.

But if navigating these different options seems overwhelming, Eat This, Not That! Is here to help you out. The only helpful thing is making little adjustments to one's lifestyle. These small steps may help one reduce calorie intake, improve diet, and establish a healthy foundation. We have arranged a list of some of the finest and most straightforward pointers to aid you in losing those extra pounds and keeping the weight off permanently.

CHAPTER 1

PRACTICE GOOD CONSUMING HABIT

if you were told you that you could maintain the weight you want even though you could keep eating all the things you love? You may think we're insane, but if you asked us, we'd tell you that this is the path of least resistance. Think back to the last time you tried to follow a low-carb diet. How long did it take you before you gave up and bought a pizza instead? We are willing to gamble that it happened far sooner than you are ready to accept it did. The reason for this is that rather than focusing on developing good eating habits, you are attempting to alter the foods that you consume. You see, the reason why losing those first few pounds is so challenging is that the majority of weight-loss procedures start by removing things from your diet. This is one of the reasons why dropping those first few pounds is so difficult. Even while this makes perfect sense, adding one significant dietary change on top of another significant nutritional change is not only exhausting but also has the potential to make you feel deprived and depressed. Because of this, you could initially see weight loss, but the weight may quickly return to its previous level.This list is not like any other in that regard. These suggestions will help you improve the way you eat, not the foods you consume. That's fine, go ahead and chow down on that pizza! Just make sure that you are seated at the dinner table, that the time is around 6:30, and that you are pausing between meals to engage in conversation with your family. You will quickly discover that making a few simple tweaks to your late-night pizza binges while you're alone may pay off and help you keep the weight off in the long term. If you adopt just a handful of these more nutritious eating practices, you'll be able to shed those extra ten pounds in no time!

Don't eat after 9 pm.

It's not true that your metabolism will begin to slow down when you reach this age; it's just a myth about food. Research published in the journal Appetite found that those who eat late at night are more likely to put on weight than those who get up early to take advantage of early bird specials. This was shown to be the issue when comparing the two groups likelihood of gaining weight. It's not because they don't burn those calories as fast; it's because night owls are more prone to binge eat (after starving themselves since lunch) and then choose unhealthy foods that are heavy in sugar and fat to put in their growling bellies quickly. This causes them to gain weight. Not only can these high-energy meals cause you to gain weight, but many of them will also make it more difficult for you to go to sleep at night. And in case you are bot aware, one of the solutions to the question of how to lose ten pounds is to increase the amount of sleep you receive each night.

Reward yourself and console yourself without the use of food.

The key to a successful strategy to lose weight is to set objectives for yourself and work toward achieving them. And although it's true that any weight reduction, even one pound, is cause for celebration, it doesn't mean you should reward yourself by indulging in your go-to comfort food once you reach your goal weight. It would help if you instead made an effort to reward yourself in ways that do not include food, such as purchasing a new exercise tank for yourself, spending on a fitness class, or going to the movies with your friends. Eliminating the association between eating and feeling a certain way will make it simpler to make healthier food choices in the future.

Remove any potential sources of distraction while eating.

It's time to put an end, for good, to the practice of eating in front of the television; according to the findings of research titled "Meal Quality and Preference," those who listened to music via headphones while eating consumed noticeably more of the same food when compared to individuals who were not engaged in musical activity.

Specialists have shown that keeping your mind occupied as you eat might prevent some satiety signals from signaling to your brain that you have consumed enough food to satisfy your hunger. Therefore, if you are trying to lose weight, one of the finest things you can do is to follow one of our top weight loss ideas and put your TV remote or Spotify playlist on pause while you eat.

Sit down

We are fine for walking meetings, as long as they are not lunch meetings.

Walking meetings are a great idea. This is because research has shown that those who stand while chewing end up gorging themselves with thirty percent more food during their subsequent meal compared to those who sit. Researchers hypothesize that this is due to the fact that our bodies
unconsciously see a meal that is served at a particular time as a "fake meal," which prompts us to consume additional food later in the day.

Keep eating and sleeping separately in your bedroom at all times.

There was a correlation between having a television in the bedroom and having a lower amount of overall sleep duration, according to a study published in the journal Sleep Medicine. Not only will watching tv in bed hinder you from obtaining a restful night's sleep (which, in case you weren't aware, is one of the most important guidelines for losing weight), but eating in bed will also prevent you from losing weight. Your brain and body may be trained to equate getting under the covers with sleep if you make your bedroom your designated sleeping space. This will make it much simpler for you to get some shut-eye when you need it.

Consider whether or not you are, in fact, hungry.

You don't need to get extra-large popcorn just because you're going to attend a movie, even if you are planning on doing so. The same may be said for the food that was consumed during the morning meeting but was not eaten and has been deposited in the breakroom. It is not necessary to consume food just because you do not have to pay for it or because you are experiencing feelings of boredom. Always question yourself, "Am I genuinely hungry?" whenever you find yourself in the presence of food that tempts you. Put yourself to the test by downing a cup of water and giving yourself ten

minutes to think about it. According to research that was published in Physiology and Behavior, almost sixty percent of the time, individuals react improperly to their thirst by eating rather than drinking. It's one of the many reasons why you're starving all the time.
Well, this is the first day of the rest of your life, as we are certain that our detailed weight reduction guide will explain to you the fundamentals of weight training, map out a plan for your success, and provide you with actionable advice for fine-tuning your workout routine.

Chapter 2

WEIGHT LOSS TIPS

How Exactly Does Weight Loss Occur?
(Reduce your intake of calorie and nincrease your physical activity)

Reducing caloric intake combined with increasing energy expenditure is the fundamental mechanism behind weight loss.Dietary restraint is the key to weight loss.Get moving more often.You may either focus on one method, like dieting or mix the two, like exercising more.

Say, for instance, that you need to consume 2,000 calories daily to stay the same weight. If you consume 1,500 calories daily, you will have a deficit of 500 calories per day, equivalent to losing around 1 pound every week.

Alternately, you might keep eating 2,000 calories daily and increase your activity level to burn more than 200 more calories per day by walking and other means.

Step 1: Determine Your Daily Maintenance Calorie Needs

How many calories you need to eat daily to stay current weight may be easily determined using online calorie calculators. You may also maintain your current weight for a week by consuming the same number of daily calories.

Check your weight at the start and end of the week to see whether it has changed. The degree to which these numbers change or remain unchanged will tell you whether you are making progress toward your goal or falling short.

Step 2:Tracking calories and evaluating eating patterns

Second, if you're trying to lose weight, keeping a food diary using an app like MyFitnessPal may be a big help. If it is more convenient, you may keep a physical notebook to record your calorie intake and expenditure. Choose wisely so that you have a better chance of sticking with it.

Many individuals don't realize that they're eating too much, underestimating their caloric intake by as much as 40 per cent. It is possible to wipe out your deficit if you are one of the many individuals who fail to enter all their food while keeping track of calories.

Don't forget to log food and drink as you go. It's possible to consume 103 calories only from one can of beer. Because 500 calories are so low, careful monitoring is essential.

Most Persons overestimate the number of calories they burn while exercising, which leads to unhealthy binge eating. The data from fitness trackers and smartwatches won't be perfect, which might lead you to overeat.

Step 3:Examine your routine

Determine what time of day you eat the most by keeping a notc of your eating habits. Some folks have nighttime cravings for sweets, while others are persistent all-day snackers. When do you want to reward yourself? How about you? Do you go for the salty or sweet options? What

kinds of nutritious meals do you already like to eat?
The next step is to discover the nutritious foods you currently love and gradually swap them out for bad ones. I think you're a fan of peanut butter and sweet fruits; if so, try spreading some over apple slices and enjoying them in place of a cupcake.

Aim for healthy eating at least 80% of the time, and treat yourself 20% of the time. It's easy to make little changes, such as swapping out a few snacks, that may lead to larger changes, such as swapping out fast food for home-cooked meals. Modifying your routine slowly is a crucial first step for anybody looking to lose weight, as it will help you dodge feeling overwhelmed or discouraged.

Step 4:Create a calorie deficit

Knowing your maintenance calorie needs and being aware of your favourite unhealthy foods makes losing weight easy. If so, at least try to curb your need to constantly munch. Compared to maintenance calorie needs, a shortfall of 500 calories per day results in a loss of around 1 pound.

Step 5:Cut Back on Sugar and Processed Foods

When you eat sugar, you want more sugar. Do we agree? Almost everything you purchase at the grocery store, even fruit drinks, will have added sugar, which is extremely addictive since it stimulates the brain's pleasure centres.

Some people have found that giving up all added sugar and eating naturally sweet foods like fruits is the most effective method to curb sugar cravings and shed pounds. People who have undertaken "30-day weight reduction challenges" attest that doing so may help them permanently abstain from sugar by acclimating their brain to a world without it.

If you're trying to lose weight, it's best to steer clear of diet Coke and other sugar-free beverages since they might stimulate the same areas of the brain and make you desire real sugar.

White bread, white rice, white flour, etc., all have a high glycemic index, which means eating them will produce an insulin rise and subsequent hunger pains. It would help if you tried to limit your intake of these since they also cause water retention and abdominal swelling.

Step 6: Stay Hydrated and Cut Back on Other Liquid Calories

Sixty per cent of the time, rather than quenching our thirst, we reach for food. Maintaining a constant water intake and carrying a water bottle may help you shed pounds. If you drink more water, your body won't have as much of a need to cling to whatever fluids it comes into contact with, and you won't seem as puffy and swollen as you would otherwise before dieting.

Dehydration may interfere with your body's ability to regulate temperature and slow down your recovery time after a workout, making it all the more crucial that you stay hydrated. Keep hydrated by taking sips of water before, after, and even while you work out.

In addition, consuming at least half a litre of water 30 minutes before a meal may aid in satiety and food intake control, leading to decreased food consumption and weight loss. People who follow this advice often see an average weight loss of 44% greater than those who don't!

Avoid sugary beverages and fruit juices if you need to stay hydrated. Calories in liquid form are particularly insidious and may sabotage your diet and weight reduction efforts. The 140 calories in a can of ordinary Coke are nearly as much as a full dinner, so drinking only two cans daily is already quite a lot.As with other commercially available beverages, fruit juices are high in sugar but provide none of the beneficial fibre that comes with eating whole fruits. Fruit-infused water is a tasty alternative to sugary fruit drinks and sodas, plus it's better for your digestive system.

Step 7:Move more

Now that you know what to eat to kick-start your weight loss let's talk about the other half of the equation: increasing your physical activity.

You can exercise more without devoting weekly hours to the gym if you move about more. Non-Exercise Activity

Thermogenesis (NEAT) is the process of spending calories on breathing, digesting, and other involuntary processes by just living your regular life, and any low-intensity motions or exercise facilitates it. So, if you want to burn more calories overall, increasing your daily step count can help you achieve that goal even while you sleep.

Taking the stairs instead of the elevator, parking further away, grocery shopping instead of ordering in, doing household duties like cleaning, etc., are all great examples of baby steps in the right direction. To reduce weight, you may start with these adjustments before thinking about changing your diet.

Incorporating Walking into Your Exercise Routine

A 30-minute to an hour-long stroll is a great way to get in some exercise even if you don't have access to a gym, can't perform moderate or high-intensity exercise, or don't have much time to take up sports.

You may take a walk first thing in the morning, last thing at night, or break it up into three 10- to 20-minute segments throughout the day to keep yourself energized. If that seems too much, take a few 5-minute walks whenever convenient and work up to 10- to 20-minute walks.

Performing Exercises with a Rapid Pace and Depth Is "not having time" an excuse you often use for not working out? We understand that it may be difficult for people to carve out even an hour or two each week for physical activity; after a long day at the office, all you want to do is kick back and unwind. If you want to improve your fitness and lose weight more quickly, try doing more short, high-intensity exercises. High-intensity interval training (HIIT) involves alternating periods of high effort with periods of lower intensity to get the desired results. High-intensity interval training (HIIT) is a short-duration exercise strategy that has increased fat-burning by up to 28.5% compared to moderate exercise.

Regular moderate-intensity exercise is also a fantastic choice for weight reduction if you can't undertake HIIT for medical reasons or because you don't find it appealing. High-intensity exercise is dangerous for those with cardiac problems.

You may become in shape by walking, running, and dancing. Follow your passions and have a good time!

Do Weightlifting

Working out weights is the best way to burn fat, build muscle, and become stronger. However, you need not worry about being bulky if that is not your goal since bodybuilders' extreme diets and training regimens with highly muscled bodies are tough to imitate.

You will develop a strong, lean physique that is also attractive. Building muscle allows you to consume more without adding extra fat since it takes more energy to break down one pound of muscle than one pound of fat.

Exercise tips

You may also move your body by dancing, swimming, hiking, cycling, or anything else you like. Get into a routine or pick up an activity you may enjoy for the rest of your life that you will find rewarding.

Getting more active should be pleasurable, so don't stress too much. If you follow these guidelines, you can maintain your motivation and push through any barriers standing in your way.

Step 1-Find an activity you like; it doesn't matter how much weight you lose or how many abs and muscles you build. Suppose you hate doing exercise and quit after a few sessions.

Find anything you love doing, like weightlifting, swimming, jogging, Zumba, yoga, or anything else, and stick with it for lifetime

Step 2-If you have never worked out, begin with a little program. Walks and light, low-intensity activities are great places to begin. This rule of thumb is universal; if you've never done HIIT before, do it for no more than 5 minutes at a time. Start with three exercises, three times a week, for weight training. Every action counts!

Step 3-Put an end to thinking that you have to go all out right immediately; any additional action is better than none. Discipline is what gets you the outcomes you want, not momentary motivation. You haven't veered off course if for whatever reason, you can only run for five minutes instead of 10 or if you can't lift as much weight as you usually do. Keep working to improve your performance every day.

Step 4-The fourth strategy is to "stack" good habits by incorporating physical activity into pre-existing routines. Did you know that the average American spends an hour a night watching Netflix? Afterwards, walk around the block or do some squats in your living room! The term "habit stacking" refers to linking a new habit with an existing one to facilitate its development. Methods for shedding those extra pounds

Chapter 3

SUCCESSFUL WEIGHT LOSS TIPS

Everyone wants to look their best. Positivity and pride are increased as a result. Unfortunately, as we age, our bodies will alter significantly. As we grow older our metabolism naturally slows, making weight loss incredibly challenging for many of us. Noting that reducing weight is about more than simply avoiding bad meals is crucial. It is always consistent with eating healthily and exercising regularly.

Self-control and perseverance can help you stick to your diet and see results. Here are the 10 most important and optimal dietary guidelines for weight loss.

1. Making your diet more efficient begins with a well-thought-out strategy

It's onyou to decide which eating routine you will commit to. It's best to plan your meals for the week and make a shopping list of everything you'll need before the week begins.

2. Don't go without eating

Skipping meals is not necessary for weight loss, despite popular belief. Regular eating is very recommended. Breakfast is the day's most important meal; thus, you should never miss it. Additionally, eating smaller meals 5-6 times a day assists your body in performing more effectively throughout the day. Regular meals help maintain healthy blood sugar and brisk fat-burning rate.

3. Avoid eating processed foods

The prevalence of processed food in our culture is undeniable. They don't need much time in the kitchen, and sometimes you can even eat them straight from the package. You may save time and effort, but ultimately you'll be setting yourself up for a lifetime of poor health if you rely on these meals. Many processed meals include unhealthy levels of salt, fat, and sugar that prevent you from losing weight. Make an effort to eat more whole, fresh meals, preferably ones you have prepared yourself.

4. Opt for Good Fats

You probably already know that certain fats are good for you. Be careful to read the nutrition labels when selecting items from the shelves so you can control the quantity and kind of fats you consume. Saturated and trans fats are unhealthy fats that contribute to high cholesterol levels. Consuming healthy fats, such as mono and polysaturated fats, will have the opposite impact and bring down your unhealthy cholesterol levels. Many foods, like avocados, cheese, and almonds, contain beneficial fats.

5. Try to Eat a Lot of Protein-Rich Foods

Every cell in our body relies on protein. Therefore we need a good supply of it every day. Its unique properties include mending damaged cells, developing bones and muscles, and speeding up recovery time after strenuous exercise. Some amino acids also help you shed pounds. Complete proteins may be found in whey, casein, egg whites, and nuts, among other foods. You may also benefit from protein powders and protein bars.

6. Be Aware of Your Calorie Intake
Increase your calorie intake if gaining muscle is your goal, but reduce your intake if weight loss is your primary objective. Put on weight if you use more calories than you lose. Beverages, including soft drinks, juices, and other similar liquids, are often quite rich in calories and should be avoided if possible. Water is the optimal fluid of choice. You may also get creative with black coffee or unsweetened tea.

7. Consume Enough Water Before Meals
We must remember to always consume enough water and other fluids daily. Similarly, some people advocate drinking water before eating. You may increase the calories you burn by around a few after drinking water before a meal. This effect can last two hours or less. Drinking

half a litre of water an hour before meals have been shown in studies to help dieters consume fewer calories and lose up to 44% more weight than those who don't.

8. Take Intermittent Fasting Into Account
It's likely that if you spend much time online or on social media, you've heard of the diet strategy known as intermittent fasting. You'll skip meals or eat very little to reduce calories on this diet. There is evidence that following a diet may help people lose weight, gain muscle, and become more insulin sensitive. Whether you're not sure if this kind of diet is right for you and your health situation, however, it's best to talk to a professional.

9. Refrain from Eating Sweets
This rule seems to explain itself, I suppose. Most everyday items have extra sugar added to them, contributing to the obesity, diabetes, and cardiovascular disease epidemic. Sugar is a

major contributor to excess body fat, so if you want to slim down, you should limit your intake of sweets and other processed foods. Dietary progress will be hindered at best.

10.Eat Off of More Plates

Another unusual suggestion that turns out to be useful. It's recommended that smaller plates be used while cooking for a group. Reduced portion sizes correspond to smaller plates. Less food eaten at once means less calorie and fat consumption. However, if you are committed to making positive changes in your life, you may master the art of self-restraint and go on the path to a healthier diet and way of life.

Chapter 4

STAY POSITIVE

Positivity is key to losing weight.

Most individuals are unaware that practically any diet may help you lose weight. The trick to losing weight, regardless of the diet you choose, is whether or not your mindset is in the proper place. A positive outlook might help you remain motivated when tempted to stray from your weight-loss plan and make it simpler to stick with.

You're setting yourself for failure from the start if you convince yourself that your weight-loss program will be challenging, dull, or that you'll feel deprived.

The following factors are common motivators for weight loss:

- They don't like the size or form of their bodies, and they think decreasing weight would make them look and feel better about their bodies.

- They want to look well in an outfit for a big event or trip.
- They attempt to manage a medical condition, lessen discomfort, or enhance their health.
- The issue is that the first two outside factors are often temporary remedies based on negativity. Short-lived motivation like this might make you feel worse than you did before.

It might be far more motivating to concentrate on how you feel when you make good decisions that support long-term health. The finest weight-reduction programs include healthy lifestyle decisions that lead to long-term benefits in weight loss and health.

The following mental advice may boost your efforts to lose weight:

Set realistic objectives. One day at a time is the key to long-term weight reduction. Huge objectives, such as "I want to drop 30 pounds in two months," may be excessively demanding. When you concentrate on breaking down a big objective into smaller stages, it's more possible, feasible, and simpler to establish long-lasting habits. Before adopting the next healthy habit, you may start by giving up all beverages with added sugar for a week and replacing them with water.

Be thankful for your attitude. Making a list of the things you are grateful for can improve your mental well-being and disposition, whether you write them down, say them out loud, or think about them. Use this method at the beginning and end of each day and before exercising.

Do not use the scale

if possible. Although little daily weight swings are common, obsessing over the scale is unhealthy. There are other methods to monitor your progress if the number on the scale gives you anxiety, such as observing how your clothing fits and measuring your body circumference.

Use optimistic visualization. Even though it may seem woo-woo, seeing yourself at your ideal weight might help you stay motivated and remind you why you began on the days when you'd rather miss a workout or have a cheat meal. You may conquer obstacles in the kitchen and the gym with its assistance. You can't perform a set of push-ups, or you don't like kale, so what gives? Watch how your results change when you switch out the negatives (I don't, I can't) with positive statements!

Celebrate your accomplishments

Create a list of non-food activities you'd want to partake in when you accomplish your large and small objectives rather than rewarding yourself with snacks and unhealthy meals! Be happy with your achievements!

Your weight-loss journey involves your thinking just as much as food and activity. Be aware of your triggers, refrain from critical self-talk, and always remember to give yourself credit. With this optimistic mindset, you'll discover that losing weight is easier.

www.ingramcontent.com/pod-product-compliance
Lightning Source LLC
LaVergne TN
LVHW052111160826
845678LV00015B/3486

* 9 7 9 8 3 5 1 9 5 9 3 8 2 *